NATURAL CURES
FOR PERFECT
HEALTH!

Jesus Christ Will Cure You,

But The Doctors Won't

By: Shelly Jenkins, BSN, RN

NATURAL CURES FOR PERFECT HEALTH!
Jesus Christ Will Cure You, But The Doctor Won't

Copyright © 2017 Shelly Jenkins, BSN, RN

ISBN-13: 978-1544223810

ISBN-10: 1544223811

Printed in the United States of America.

Kingdom Consulting and Publishing

TABLE OF CONTENTS:

Dedication

To Stephanie, Aniya and Aaron, my inspiration for staying well.

After you read this book if you feel like I've provided you with quality content and valuable information would you do me a HUGE favor please? I would appreciate it if you would write me a great five star customer review for this book on Amazon. Hopefully our paths will cross at some point in our lives and we can meet each other in person. I pray that you will be blessed with perfect health, abundant wealth and never ending happiness! Feel free to contact me at the email address below. God bless you!

Shellyjenkins13@gmail.co

Chapter One:

What is Divine Health?

"The Kingdom of God is like a treasure…." Jesus said in Matthew 13:44, "hidden in a field for years and then accidently found by a trespasser. The finder is ecstatic- what a find!—and proceeds to sell everything he owns to raise money and buy that field."

If you look at this scripture carefully, you will see that Jesus is giving us a list of prerequisites on what it takes to get into His health care system. The trespasser finds it "by accident". He throws away the other way of living by selling everything he owns. Then he is willing to go through a process (raises money) to buy the field, moving to live in a new place because now he has nothing to go back to. He is starting a new way of life.

Anything having to do with the Kingdom of God is way better. It's about a quality standard. God is waiting for someone to believe and agree with him so he can show us *His* standards. God's standards are higher than ours. And he never lowers them for us. So we must grow up to his standards. After all, He is the King right? And if we are his children, then what do you suspect he wants for us. THE BEST.

In fact, he wants it for all of us. He went through great trouble to pay for us to have it, 39 stripes I recall (therefore it is no cost or charge for you). We don't pay for health in God's system, it's not about money to get it like the earth cursed system requires. It's an inheritance.

"I have a Health Care System........." he told me one day. I feel that when he gave me this revelation, he was going somewhere with this and wanted me to go there too.

"What! What do you mean?? Why are you just now telling me this, I asked? I have spent a career working in the medical field. I could have used this knowledge years ago. Why did you wait to tell me this now?" Silence, then "Because you wouldn't have believed it," He replied. Duh, but he was right. For me it was a hidden treasure.

He has a health care system? I started to think and I began to recall. Jesus did heal many people. For years, I read about the stories in the bible. There were miraculous healings: lame, deaf and mute people

walking and talking and hearing
again. Tough stuff happening,
curses from leprosy and
epilepsy-gone. Other problems
like female problems, fevers,
(the common stuff). Still others
who got restoration from mania
and mental illness (the real stuff)
and deformities (the ugly stuff).
Even resurrection from the
Dead! (The "HE DID WHAT?!"
stuff).

Jesus was a one man
health care system. He was
going around healing everyone
of everything, the crowds
poured in. Now this lead to him
eventually being killed, even

thought people saw the results were REAL.

But what about a lifestyle of healing, being healed every single day, from every single thing. A system....that's not the same as or doesn't define a one day miracle. Jesus didn't have people who came back again with a healing that "didn't work." No frequent flyers or medical records. To "prosper and be in good health even as your soul prospers", 3 John 1:2. It's the real thing y'all. Oh, I know accidents occur and yes people get sick but I do think we should take God at his Word and say there *shouldn't* be anything wrong with me.

How many people can say that today? We know that the current health care system is so complex and costly that no solution seems to work, no matter who tries to solve it. With all its achievements, advancements and technological wonders, it still is mediocre at best. Especially compared to what Jesus did.

But God has a **health care system**? A "I can stay well system"? He has *a way* of taking care of our health? It **would** be difficulty to serve Him if I'm sick. Let's see, all my life I have used the earth cursed system (as my pastor refers to it) of health care: had to make appointments, co-pays, and deductibles. I've had to call and cancel or "get the $25 you didn't call us so we could have given your appointment to someone else" charge. I've waited in lines, and waiting on the line and been hung up on. I've been asked to reschedule or asked to wait for weeks. I've been told we don't take new patients and we don't take that insurance and even we don't take you without any insurance. I've watched advertisement stating a medication has more side effects than it cures and antibiotics that are being given away free.

One day I got so mad at a doctor's office that I took the sign-in sheet off the clip board just to show them that they were not always in charge! It got real interesting in that waiting room full of people on the old "first come, first serve basis". It took them 30 minutes to figure out the sheet was really gone! Okay, I couldn't help myself, I was angry. You gotta admit that was pretty creative. They got that sign in sheet back when they started being nice to me. I got respect after that.

Now don't get me wrong, any system is better than no system. But what God was saying was there are two systems going on here, The Kingdom of God and the system of the earth for health. They both have different results too. Trust me, I know. Be honest, you know that too.

What is God's health care system? What does "Divine Health" look like I wondered? Today, I don't believe God wants us just to get healed but to walk in "Divine Health". When the children of Israel left from Egypt, God told them to eat a specific meal. And then they left the next day "no feeble among them" Psalms 105:37. That was about receiving divine health. No one was sick for the trip to the Promise Land. They needed to be well to make that trip which was God's will for them. But we have fallen far short of that cry today. And why is that?

First I think, we have relied upon the wrong system for the wrong things. We have put our trust in the earth cursed system and have looked to its standards of health. We've trusted it for answers.

Now some have turned to God for His Will, but then are using the earth cursed system's

ways to get health. We pay for it and then say just give it to me or give me a pill or quick answer NOW, for example. We don't let faith make a payment and then allow God, effort, and time to reveal the answers. We have relied upon prayer only to wait afterward for "something to happen" with no subsequent action. We haven't understood an important concept, the "our part concept", so we miss the blessing. We think that there is no real action required...on our behalf. We have asked but not received because we wait on God and His wonders to perform, to do what only he can do best. We want Him to do it all. But then nothing happens. Why we ask? So then we start to sink. We never believe he will do anything or we believe he will but we don't know when. We just don't think it will happen for us. Meanwhile, we suffer.

I think it's because we don't afterward "take up our bed and walk" like Jesus said. We don't get up and start to do what WE can, our part. A faith action. **We** have to do the "walking". When we work with God not wait on God for action, his results manifest.

I mean think about it. If you had been sick for such a very long time and then someone tells you to just get up and start to walk, it *would* be kinda crazy to think that could just happen. Most of us would not even have tried. Or maybe some of us could not be able to fathom what walking would be like for us. We don't know just how much effort it will take after being debilitated for so long. It would take a miracle we think. But we must try, even if we can only take one step that first day.

It is a frightening thought to come out of your Egypt, like Israel did, and go out into the desert where you have not gone before. Especially if you don't understand how God will provide for you and what he might ask you to do. Even though we asked him for freedom, we really don't know what it will mean, what it will look like, where it will take us, and what it will require. Well, it will require faith.

Chapter Two:

Faith

"But without faith it is impossible to please him: for he that cometh to God must believe that he is, and that he is a rewarder of them that diligently seek him, Hebrews 11:6. This concept of faith in Christianity always perplexed me. Faith has substance because it is of the supernatural and it is a life force. Everything from God has life then substance. But substance doesn't show up here. When it shows up here it is called manifestation, but until it does show up it's called faith?? So confusing!!

As I mentioned before, because I am guilty of it myself, I thought you pray and then wait for God to do something you asked. I never thought to apply this, to use this faith concept to my health. I found it worked the other way around. I act first, then God acts. An example of those who acted on faith as commanded and got healing were the 10 lepers in Luke 17:14. Jesus commanded them to go to the priest and "as they went" they received their healing. But they did have to take his word and rise up and go to the priest to get a manifestation of healing. So did the man at the pool of Bethesda who was told rise, take up you bed and walk. Mark2:11. They followed his instructions exactly.

But God started to show me that he wanted me to believe for an even higher standard of health, divine health. Health in which I could play an active part and get His results permanently. A systematic way to have health. He showed me that when Jesus said, "It is finished," on the cross, he meant that the way and the power for health is now in my court. I didn't have to ask for it anymore. I just had to follow the rules of the Kingdom of God and it would manifest in my life. It's a benefit of Kingdom living or citizenship. It's a principle of the Kingdom not to catch a fish just to eat for a day but to learn to fish and eat for a lifetime.

Like Dorothy in the Wizard of Oz, you're already standing in the shoes honey! (I love that movie so I'll use this as an example). Shoes, symbolically speaking, were the source of power. Yes, she already had the power and I already have the power. "Everything I need pertaining unto life and godliness", 2 Peter 1:3 is on the inside of me. Course Dorothy found that out like I did, at the end of the movie, ha ha! It's not really the shoes it's who I am, walking in the shoes.

Furthermore, Dorothy had to get mad and destitute to use the power most times, curls bouncing and all! She was even using the power subconsciously when she recruited her friends through the power of love and compassion, and each time she faced the wicked witch and her schemes. She didn't realize it. She was frustrated because like me, I'm told what I'm supposed to have but don't know how to use that power. But think about it, she had to know she didn't get those shoes for nothing the first day she stood in them. She was even warned, whatever you do, "DO NOT TAKE THEM OFF!" Even if just subconsciously, she should have had gut feelings that they were of great value, right? I liked the scene when the witch tried to touch them and electricity emanated from them! Woo whoa, shocking!!

This story was a good object lesson for me, a visual if you will. Yes, Dorothy just didn't know how much she was really given that day. Most of all she didn't know that she didn't need a Wizard to help her! That's how we see doctors and the medical field, the earth cursed health care system I think. They are the great and powerful Oz. People run to them like they really are. Putting so much faith and demand on them for their services, even unto death….But in God's reality we have everything we need right now, so how can we use it? How do we make the connection? Who will we put our trust in?

Now like Hebrews 11 this is my faith chapter. Faith works like this, I have to make the first move. God always tells me "Shelly, I'm waiting on you." You know what gets me now? How people can be in a sinking ship, not recognizing something is wrong and not ask God for help and guidance, like the listing Titanic. Then they don't take help when it comes, like the half-filled lifeboat. Sometimes people don't recognize when God shows up. How sad is that? If nothing else, we should be trying to establish a stronger "signal or uplink" to God through their actions. But instead, its "God you're break up, you're breaking up!"

Yesterday a lady was brought into my office by her boss having chest pain. She said she had already been to the doctor who had run tests and told her everything was ok. We called her doctor and no one answered. We waited and called again. They told her to go to the urgent care clinic next door at 5:30 in the evening. She discussed with me some life style changes and mentioned a few things she had done but wasn't open to anything else. I asked had she prayed for guidance. She looked a bit surprised and said no, I haven't. The pain continued as she kept grabbing her chest. Her vital signs were okay so I asked her to call her relative to take her to the doctor or I need to call a squad. She wouldn't call saying her sister overreacts. She wouldn't go to the hospital. So all I could do was check the AED to make sure it was working. Go figure.

Now me, when my signal to God is getting weak, I'm doing something I shouldn't be doing or doing too much (the unimportant). I'm not always willing to do some things but many times my success is contingent on what I *am* willing to do.

I heard a pastor say that our culture is a culture heavily dependent on mood and mind altering agents (Pharmacia). Anything that makes us feel good and numbs us to the adversities of life. So as a result I can't feel anything, so I won't *do* anything.

When I threw my medications in my drawer, it was an act of faith. I had finally got good and tired of the earth cursed system. Ok I said, it's you and me now God (and I didn't know what or how it was going to happen). All the reasons why I started taking that stuff in the first place started coming back. Guess who was now well motivated and willing to seek God for help? I screamed for it, I was not used to really experiencing my emotions and pain since I would quickly anesthetize them. I had to start learning to deal with them immediately (with the help of God, His grace and His power). That was frightening at first. But using THAT kind of faith, He started showing me what He wanted me to do.

Some barriers to this process are fear and pride. "I'm sckared!" Good old fear. I'm not going to do that, what will people think? Good old pride. Or that seems stupid. Or I'd have to humble myself and that's humiliating! Good old, well crazzzzy! I'm not going to eat vegetables while you guys eat pizza.

But in the Kingdom of God there's one thing you can't be, a coward. And another, a know it all. There's serious work to be done if the proverbial ball is in your court. In fact, each day counts.

I remember when I was a kid; there were headlines in the news about the "race to space". We were trying to beat the Russians to the moon. They got out there in space faster than we did, but we were afraid of what they would do with that knowledge and position so we had to get in the fight. It was a matter of survival. We didn't know what they would do next?

That is how it works with the earth cursed system. If we don't get on top of it, it will get on top of us. We have to make even every second count. I think about this as I write this book. I could have been watching TV. But people need help. And when they are willing and ready, it needs to be there. That's part of God's Health Care System. The information will be there to help you when you seek it.

Chapter Three:

What Has God Promised?

I think it is fundamental to know what to expect from God by knowing what His Word really says. I looked at what the Word of God tells us. Keep in mind that God wouldn't be healing all those people if he didn't want us well. His desire is for you to "have life, and life more abundantly", John 10:10.

Twice God said in Deuteronomy 28 that if we listen to him and observe his commandments that he will set us upon high in many areas of life. Specifically in Psalms 103:2-

3 He says to praise Him and don't forget his benefits—He heals all our diseases. All meaning all. The same power that gave us salvation and forgiveness heals our bodies. Take a look at these scriptures in the Old Testament:

Jehovah Rapha means he is "The LORD that heals." Exodus 15:26.

Exodus 23:25 Worship the Lord your God, and His blessings will be on your food and water. I will take away sickness from among you.

In the message bible:

2 Chronicles 7:14 says that if "my people, my God-defined people, respond by humbling themselves, praying seeking my presence, and turning their backs on their wicked lives, I'll be there ready for you: I'll listen from heaven, forgive their sins, and restore their land to health."

"Those who discover these words live, really live; body and soul, they're bursting with health". Proverbs 4:22

"Listen for God's voice in everything you do, everywhere you go; he's the one who will keep you on track. Don't assume that you know it all. Run to God. Run from evil! Your body will glow with health, your very bones will vibrate with life" Proverb 3:6-8.

Job 2:5 "But what do you think would happen if you reached down and took away his health?" When Satan said this he knew that Job was used to enjoying good health so much so, that if it were removed he would not be able to tolerate it.

Again in the Message Bible Psalms 41:3 says, "Whenever we're sick and in bed, God becomes our nurse, nurses us back to health." In chapter 104:15 it says "Their faces glowing with health, a people well-fed and hearty."

In the New Testament, there are a lot of people who received healing and became whole which was a gift to them to start a new way of life:

God says in 3 John 1:2 that he wants us to enjoy good health body, mind, and spirit. In Philippians 3:21 He says he changes our bodies into glorious bodies like His.

Jesus said, "and when he had called unto his twelve disciples, he gave them power against unclean spirits, to cast them out, and to heal all manner of sickness and all manner of disease. Matthew 10:1.

These scriptures from God's World show us what God's desire for our health should be. We should expect no less. We should accept no less.

Chapter Four:

Jesus Christ Or The Doctor

So what system are you using? You know, there are no doctors and nurses in the Kingdom of God. But only "apostles, prophets, evangelist, pastor and teachers, for the perfecting of the saints, for the work of the ministry, for the edifying of the body of Christ. Till we all come in the unity of the faith, and of the knowledge of the Son of God, unto a perfect man unto the measure of the stature of the fullness of Christ" (Ephesians 4:12-13).

That was all that God felt we needed. He gave us leadership, instruction, overseers and people to speak into our lives. In the book of 1 Kings 17:10-24, the widow of Zarephath got everything she needed from Elijah. She received unlimited food in a famine and the resurrection of her son who got sick and died. He was a prophet of God.

But the other system, it's a myriad of individuals who are independent of one another and not working collectively. Their purpose is not the greater good and their means is themselves. It's about dollars and cures that temporarily work then fail us. It's "pills and bills, just pills and bills (a quote from Mrs. Snow in the movie Pollyanna). Promises they can't keep to people who have spent all their money and now are just waiting to die. They hope that time won't run out before the miracle happens.

Now there are sincere people in those venues just like me. They trained hard, came to work and worked hard, went home exhausted (me personally I had calluses on my feet). They kept up expensive credentials, worked long hours and spent many a holiday without family. Overtime list was all the way down to the floor. But we just didn't know what we didn't know. So those without Christ; some system is better than no system.

So I finally thought of **not** calling my doctor, throwing all my pills in a drawer and saying "well God, it's just you and me now". Took me 30 years to get there. I couldn't handle the egotistical people, unsolved costly medical problems and the upfront copays "before you even see the water fountain" anymore. Just when I said I refuse to go to another hospital or doctor I don't care what happens, I hear this smug sounding voice say, "I have a health care system…." What? I said. He repeated it, "I have a health care system." That day changed my life and my practice. I'm glad because I had no other recourse.

As people we would rather put our trust in the earth cursed system AND get their results instead of trust in God. As a matter of fact, we don't even consider that there may even be another way of handling this situation. For me, my pride kept me from finding the hidden treasure. I was trespassing when I found it you could say. I thank God today for showing me this.

Chapter Five:

Obedience

And Samuel said, "Hath the LORD as great delight in burnt offerings and sacrifices, as in obeying the voice of the LORD. Behold, to obey is better than sacrifice, and to hearken better than the fat of rams."1 Samuel 15:22.

Now once you turn toward God for better health, obedience to what he shows you is imperative. I could not have tolerated the sleepless nights and pains in my body without being willing to do what God said after those pills were surrendered.

"But Daniel determined that he would not defile himself by eating the king's food or drinking his wine….." Daniel 1:8 in the Message Bible.

The first thing God told me to do was look at how I was treating my body, a temple of His Spirit. Over the years I had done terrible things to it. I put numerous chemicals in it, I smoked, I drank, I didn't get enough sleep, worked long hours, starved it, put junk food in it, had an accidental injury requiring stitches twice, broke bones, many infections, several surgeries. I generally was desecrating and was destroying it. It's hard to walk in divine health if we are part of the problem. We have to turn from our sinful ways. So by the time I turned to the earth cursed system, I wasn't in great shape then. After their intervention I was battle weary.

Let me reiterate, some system is better than none and it kept me until I could get to a place of desperation and faith in what God may have to offer. And let me point out that God can and sometimes does allow that other system to give us some relief but it is not His best choice for us or His Will for us.

And let me say that people know what they should be doing regarding their health. I know because they don't want to hear it again when I tell them. They hear the nagging on the inside telling them, "Quit smoking! You need more rest. You should take it easy, or you should stop taking it easy and get some work done. Go take a walk or get some exercise. Stop all that extreme exercising!" Here's the big one, "Eat this and don't eat that! Stop, don't, quit, start!" We go on ignoring Him until something

serious happens. We swear off.
Then we do it some more.

Chapter Six:

Present My Body

Romans 12:1 "Present our bodies a living sacrifice, holy and acceptable unto God which is our responsible service…… that we may prove what is the good, and acceptable, and perfect will of God."

It's a proper sacrificial offering that He said He will approve and bless. Abel made a proper sacrifice, which God said he would approved. Cain did it his way. Solomon made sacrifices to God that were approved and greatly rewarded.

Consecration (meaning to dedicate to a sacred purpose) has probably been one of the most difficult things I have done to service God and obtain divine health. But I can't by any means say it was not worth all the effort I have and continue to put into it.

In the beginning I didn't get it, especially when I did not see a lot of people around me in the Christian community doing it. Every now and then I would see someone lose weight or notice someone with a striking clear complexion. We were told to stop drinking or smoking or eating poorly. For me it was not a reality. Usually, when there are events at church, I am tempted more than usual by the food I see being served.

Me myself, I was raised by a sugar addict. However, my father ate well. Today he is 90 years old. My mom died of diabetes and cancer. By being around my mom most of the time, guess what I learned to enjoy with no boundaries? When the health problems started, I didn't know where to start. I began to realize I would have many of the health problems that my patients had. I knew one thing: I didn't want to go down like that.

"Present your bodies a living sacrifice, holy and acceptable unto God which is our responsible service" Romans 12:1.

I began a slow and tedious process of confronting my problems with my body. I stopped using drugs, alcohol (thank God I didn't go as far down the paths some of my college buddies did) and fought my way out of that terrible nicotine habit (I wish I never started that fatal cool) which took 5 years. I started to tackle the food issue mainly because of the gastrointestinal problems I had all my life. I would be in the

ER as a teenager rolling around on their stretchers in pain. They had to run IV antacid medication in my arm, just to calm down my heartburn. I was always having stomach pain, then an ulcer. That was highly motivating.

I could not have done it without the power of God. He showed me the power of abstinence, first by showing me I was lactose intolerant. The knowledge to start abstaining from milk, which I drank by the gallons, was the first miracle I received. Even though when I grew up school children are given milk daily (still are), so I never questioned that something which was being promoted for good health was killing me. Once I did abstain, for the first time in life, my digestive system calmed down. I didn't know a person could feel like that.

Another problem that was becoming debilitating was stiffness in my joints. I thought it was due to the cold Midwest climate of Chicago but it wasn't. It was arthritis developing due to my gluten intolerance. I found out purely by accident when I was having trouble with my knee because of a torn ACL. A lady I heard talking said she had been so overweight, that she had no more cartilage left in her knees. Her bones would rub together and that was very painful. But she was abstaining from wheat and all her pain was gone. Well I knew what that felt like, so I tried it. Later I was to have the allergy to gluten confirmed by an integrative medicine doctor. He told me I had Celiac Disease and that I would need to abstain from wheat products. It stopped the pain and stiffness in 2 months. It probably took that long for all the wheat I binged on, through breads (my tranquilizers), to clear my system. I didn't really notice at first but as the next winter came, it went and I was no longer stiff.

It was amazing to me. Just think I didn't need a pill. It was good to have mobility back.

Roman 14:20 "do not destroy the work of God for the sake of food."
Message Bible

I still struggled with weight issues from an eating disorder and back pain which I thought was related to the weight. I found (when my fear of chiropractics was addressed) that I had scoliosis and that was why I had trouble with low back pain since my teen years. Today, a monthly visit has helped me. Especially numerous times when the activities I have done have pulled my back out. Like moving. It has relieved a weakness in my thigh muscle that was getting progressively worse in two days. I had stopped going for my visits for months. I then realized it wasn't the muscle, it was pressure on the nerves to the muscle. Chiropractics also increases the mobility in my neck.

When I sought God for help with the eating disorder, I did this through prayer and fasting (this was really difficult). The fasting calmed my flesh down so I could hear more clearly for guidance and instruction. God responded by sending me to people that were just like me, but who had found an answer to their eating problems. I was detoxed and I have started over with great success (see my next book on this process).

I was destroying my body for the sake of food. Not to mention what the gluten was doing to my gut. It was causing malabsorption and nobody told me that either. I keep the scripture in front of me about how the prophet Daniel "purposed in his heart" not to eat what the earth cursed system of Babylon ate. He made that commitment up front. He had been trained in the Word of God what to eat and what not to eat. And this was food sacrificed primarily to other gods; a god of gluttony I think. He was going to follow it. Because he made the first move, God honored it and He was given favor by the eunuch to eat the way he wanted. And he looked better because of it.

In his wisdom he knew eating that food would desecrate his body so that's how I look at it for myself. He gained a lot of benefits in the situation that he found himself in as well. Daniel survived the lion's den, and had great wisdom and health as benefits.

You know, God gave or prescribed for the Israelites a food plan for health. He knew what things would hurt their bodies. In the beginning, he told Adam what to eat too and placed it around him so he would have access to it. A physician should prescribe for his patients, what should be done to stay well. However, this doesn't happen in the earth cursed system.

Chapter Seven:

Knowledge Really Is Power

Proverbs 1:7 "the fear of the Lord is the beginning of knowledge."

"My people are destroyed for lack of knowledge." Hosea 4:6

"But be ye transformed by the renewing of your mind that you may prove what is that good, and acceptable, and perfect will of God." Romans 12:1b.

There was so much I didn't know about Kingdom Health. It was like going back to college all over again. I realized that it really was a system. There are tools, if you will, that I can use to have divine health. Faith, knowledge, trust, obedience, and discipline.

I had to pray at first to ask God to help me with what I thought was my "weight problem". I could loose and gain weight but not keep it off. I noticed with the weight came the health problems. Why couldn't I be successful? The more I tried the worse it got. That's a good time to ask for help.

He slowly started to guide me into the direction of physiology to review what I had already learned about the body, and how I could use this same knowledge to understand how Kingdom Health operated. He started to explain the questions that I had subconsciously asked back in school. Things like why are there three systems in the body to utilize energy? And how the earth cursed system uses the one for weight gain and illness and He uses the one for weight loss and health. That one way was like burning coal for fuel and the other was like using natural gas, a cleaner and more efficient fuel.

This started to set in motion for me a series of thought processes that led me to a better way of understanding why people are sick and why they are well. I know I have an advantage over people that don't have medical knowledge. But it was good to finally take what I knew before and apply it in a practical way for health care then use it as a system for divine health.

Instead of treating symptoms, God as the Great Physician, treats causes. Instead of treating just the body, he treats the soul and the spirit. Because of this approach, people are healed and experiencing total wellness. You don't just get the temporary relief you get "the whole enchilada". I'll deal with food in a minute.

When I was in college, it seemed like most lectures regarding the diseases we studied, start with the "etiology unknown". Meaning they don't know what causes the disease. I would think subconsciously to myself "They don't know what causes this? So how can we solve the problem if we don't know that?" We would study the human body, which has got to be the most incredible natural machine found on earth, and they would talk about the little they knew of how it worked.

However, discoveries were occurring all the time in "modern medicine". Things were constantly changing. We studied all those systems, with all those things that could go wrong. Disease cures were built on a lot of assumptions and speculations and some were not accurate. In nursing care, we would do interventions this way for a while then change it back to that way. It went in cycles. When we didn't understand things, we had to guess by what we would observe. When enough incidences occurred, we would come to a conclusion about how something worked or responded. Most times, intuition and experience was the most valuable thing we had going for us. So there was a movement toward evidence based practice.

But as time went on I started to realize that weight wasn't really my problem, food was. Today I believe that two things cause most diseases: something we are putting into our bodies that we shouldn't, and something we are not putting into our bodies that we that we should. The wheat and lactose situation nailed it for me.

In Deuteronomy 28, God starts out addressing what we should do and the results and then what we should not do and the results. Essentially he is saying this is a formula for living.

With God, he may have to take you through a series of events to bring you to a healthy state, but it will happen. It is what we don't know that is really causing our diseases and poor health. We don't know that we don't know. So gaining the knowledge we need is invaluable.

Health is a vast area of knowledge so doctors cannot possibly know everything to help us. But when we are sick and suffering we will trust a doctor. However, our doctors are only trained on a very limited focus of the overall system of medical science. Their perspective is through a very limited lens (not genesis of disease, or the healing of disease). They are not trained in what causes a disease, but how to manage a disease with pharmaceuticals.

The pharmaceutical and medical industry has driven the whole system and are in cahoots' together. So, as consumers, we need to know what causes diseases and also that drugs are not cures. They can manage your disease but not cure it. Not even simple stuff like heartburn, yet alone cancer.

Managing it is costing us a fortune. But there are many types of medical sciences that give us a total picture and no one science has all the answers. India's oldest system of natural medicine, Ayurvedic medicine, and traditional Chinese medicine are a few to name. Chiropractics, acupuncture, massage therapy, reflexology, are some of the other natural or "God health care" systems for health and healing.

But in the United States, these paths to healing were not well known or used until the last 20 or 30 years. Because our traditional medical system and doctors are the only medical treatment your insurance company will pay for. They have got our legislators to not allow anyone but them to practice medicine and prescribe drugs. There is not a free medical market in the USA. MDs have been driving the medical industry since the early 1900s. They are good for accidental injuries, trauma, surgery, and acute medical problems. But for chronic disease, which is what most people go to the doctor for, they can't treat you except with man-made synthetic drugs. There is a different way that we don't know about.

Here are 3 things you should know at this point about God's Health Care System; 1) The body knows how to fix itself, 2) it is endowed with a God-given intelligence, and 3) it can grow itself and wants to fix itself. God made you like that. God replicates our body through DNA coding, right? It works and grows on its own. So essentially, we are getting played like a fiddle. But thank God he is raising up a generation of physicians who practice natural medicine and who are being trained to support the body by giving it what it needs to fix itself. They don't treat diseases, they treat people. They let God be God. They give the body what it needs and let it heal itself. They are following God principles of assisting with a divine health system. These doctors call diseases by whatever deficiency you have, not names like asthma or diabetes or arthritis.

I read that there are 6 principles for naturopathic doctors:

1. First do no harm (utilize the most natural, least invasive and least toxic therapies)
2. Identify and treat the causes (look beyond the

symptoms to the
underlying cause).

3. Doctor as teacher (educate patients in the steps to achieving and maintaining health).

4. Treat the whole person (view the body as an integrated whole in all its physical and spiritual dimensions).

5. The healing power of nature (trust in the body's inherent wisdom to heal itself.

6. Prevention (focus on overall health, wellness and disease prevention). That sounds like a God

health care system!
(www.bastyr.edu).

Let's get back to our part.
Only good nutrition and
supplementation helps this (and
they don't cost like
pharmaceuticals). Today, our
bodies simply have run out of
what it needs to function. If you
cure the deficiency, it makes the
symptoms go away 100%. Again,
that sounds like a divine health
care system to me.

We need to be taught
health recovery. There are 90
essential nutrients needed. Our
body needs 60 minerals, 16
vitamins, 12 amino acids and 2
EFA's (essential fatty acids) every

day. However, we cannot get all the minerals from the food because they are no longer in the soil.

The FDA says we can only treat disease by using drugs. Then the medical field has to use diagnostic testing, imaging, surgery and chemotherapy to treat diseases. This is very invasive and costly. But there really is no such thing as a disease, just deficiencies (the something we should be eating). And inflammation due to poor nutrition (the something we shouldn't be eating). This treatment is non-invasive.

Sounds like a biblical principle, right?

The medical field says most chronic diseases are genetic or autoimmune in origin. Genetics are simply the DNA code or blue print for how tissues are produced is their argument for etiology. It is not responsible for disease. Autoimmune causes state that tissue has reversed this process or is attacking itself to cause disease. But naturopathic medicine says diseases are fixed with proper nutrients (nutrition). This is what Daniels knew and why he asked NOT to eat their food. Such diseases like asthma, diabetes, fibromyalgia, and the list goes on all due to deficiencies. You don't have a bad gene (which is God given I might add) you have an earth cursed medical system with unfortunately poorly trained doctors treating your so called disease. Their focus is not young-gevity. Their goal is not to end human suffering.

So in a divine health care system, we start out with faith and learn to trust God's guidance. We learn his new ways and become obedient and disciplined. Then he gives us physicians that teach and support his health care system.

This is the right order. But with the earth cursed system, for example, the medical industry will treat that very same arthritis with anti-inflammatory medications, pain meds, surgery, pain meds again, more anti-inflammatory medications and more surgery. But it doesn't get better. I think I would rather have the nutrition solution and supplementation.

Chapter Eight:

Discipline

So how do I get well? Start to believe God for his guidance in your particular situation. Trust his biblical principles. And most of all leave the earth cursed system!

When I embarked up this journey. I was hoping it would be fruitful. But nothing worth having ever comes easy. The things of God are free but not CHEAP. They have always required effort so being lazy (slothful) doesn't get you anywhere. I must do my part and work for what I want. Most importantly it takes discipline. I can't be all over the place, unorganized and lazy to achieve anything valuable.

Mary, the mother of Jesus, had an assignment that was quite an undertaking. She had to endure criticism, almost losing her betroth husband because in Jewish culture, to become pregnant before marriage was forbidden. I'm sure everyone else just thought she had a change in character and decided to become wayward. Notice how through angelic advice she went and stayed with her cousin Elizabeth until she gave birth to her son John. That gave her a bit of a break. She even left town by divine design and delivered her baby in Bethlehem, away from her community. It was years until she returned. But she stayed on the path. Joseph her spouse had to be told by God what his part was because he didn't believe her either.

Notice in the beginning of this book, the trespasser had to dig a hole and place the treasure in it and then go and raise money to buy the field. He couldn't sit down and hope he would just get it. If you want things from the kingdom of God I've found, you have to stay vigilant, watchful, sober minded, on duty, working, cross carrying, and productive. You will have to endure persecution too. And if you don't have a work ethic you're in trouble. You don't work, you don't eat. Gotta be like the ant.

Discipline is defined as "a way of behavior that shows a willingness to obey rules or orders, a behavior that is judged by how well one follows a set of rules or orders, instruction." God says repeatedly, especially in Deuteronomy 28 that if you hearken diligently unto his voice and observe His commandment He will respond with His part. He will set you on high or display. Like soldiers to obtain heavenly health, I will have to be disciplined in my life and affairs. This requires study, organization, willingness, and hard work.

I had to be regimented in prayer, fasting and meditation, bible reading, church attendance, participation and service. In my personal life I have had to keep grocery lists, food journals, financial records, calendars and goal posters. I had to surrender my body, the temple of His Holy Spirit to consecration and follow the practical knowledge God was leading me into. It was a commitment to God as He had made a commitment to me.

I went to church regularly and attended bible study to keep my faith going. I changed everything about my life style. When I struggled to quit those cigarettes, I had to barricade myself in the house for a week just to keep from buying them. They were on sale everywhere. I bought groceries and just didn't leave the house. I knew any block I drove down would remind me of the fact I could stop and pick some up. I sat on the porch one morning and a very strong urge to smoke came over me. I knew I was weak and

I couldn't take any challenges from my flesh at this point. I was just trying because I knew I had to do it. I didn't know how I was going to make it from one moment to the next.

As I sat there I began to feel a benevolent present in front of me. It seemed to be pleading for me to just hold on. I knew that had to be the LORD. I waited until it passed but having that presence there with me made me weep to know he cared about me that much. It distracted me from thinking about smoking and I got through it. I had tried before to quit with my husband. We both prayed and begun to abstain. The next day I noticed my whole neck area was tender to touch. I mentioned it to him and he said, "that's funny mine is too." I think God was supernaturally healing our throat areas from toxins just because we were trying to quit. And because we were a couple, what he did for me he was also doing for my husband. Got to admit I couldn't have gotten that from a doctor.

When I started working on "the food" issue I was overwhelmed. My girlfriend told me that she had given up sugar. In the back of my mind I felt I must be in some other category because that could never happen to me in this lifetime. Who could even conceive of doing something like that? Why there won't be anything left for me to eat. So I asked her "then what do you eat?" She said "I make myself chicken salad." Wow I thought. At lease that was one item. I couldn't think of anything. Do you have any idea what it took to pry sugar out of my life? Or wheat for that matter? Those were my best friends. Everything has wheat in it. Sugar too. But this diabetes thing is getting ridiculous! I didn't want to take injections like my grandmother, uncle and MY MOTHER....

Today, believe it or not it's out of my system. Stay tuned for how I did it. It's a long story but I can say this. My anxiety attacks are gone, I'm sleeping hard as a rock at night and that stubborn 15 lbs. I couldn't get off melted away. I even had to add food back into my plan to stop the weight loss. I have energy I never had before and I love the way I look! Benefits, gotta love them...this leads me to the possibilities.

Chapter Nine:

How Good Does It Get

A God health care system goes above and beyond what one would normally expect from the earth cursed system. It will deal with crisis and emergency situations in the most astounding ways.

One night I was lying in bed, fighting a terrible anxiety attack thinking I was going to just plain jump out of my skin with fear. Then I felt this presence in the room like it was standing at the end of my bed. All of a sudden, I felt something blow on me. The breath had a force that when it reached me it pressed on me and then penetrated my body. It was so peaceful that I didn't remember what had happen until I woke up the next morning. That breath of peace had put me into a sound sleep. I know now that God can address my emotional problems.

Then I started to seek God through prayer AND fasting. Let me take some time out to address this. God said if my people would humble themselves (fasting) and pray that He would honors it because it is a time that we minister or wait on or become a servant to him. Once after a three week partial fast, my granddaughter came home from a visit with her Dad and we discovered that she had stopped biting her nails. They had all grown out evenly.

I remember sharing with a girlfriend about the goodness of God and she told me that she was eating some food one day and began to choke. She was by herself and didn't have anyone to help her. From out of nowhere she said something slapped her on the back and the food came flying out of her mouth! I don't think she could have made that up. One day I started choking while swallowing a big horse pill vitamin. I could still talk but I couldn't get it out of my throat. I tried to vomiting but it wasn't in my esophagus so that didn't work. I tried the chair to do the Heimlich maneuver on myself but that didn't work either. I began to get frightened that it might eventually go into my lungs so I thought I better call the EMS. Then I heard a voice say to me "do your fingers like this…" and I immediately got a vision to put my thumb and index finger together making a birds beak. Then it said "do like this" and I got another vision to take my fingers and run them up my neck over my throat. I did it and the pill which was lying sideways like a football in my throat came right up!

But this is nothing compared to some extraordinary things that have been documented to have happened. I have been reading that God's health care system in other countries have brought healings that are unbelievable. Natural healing in countries like India have used plant herb and mineral and milk remedies that cause tissues to regenerate. Teeth start to grow back, hair to turn back black, joints, bones, ligaments, and tendons start to regenerate themselves. You look years younger when you complete this treatment.

There is research by the Russians on peptides that can cause limbs to regrow (it's on You Tube).   Fingers have been grown back, even with the nail replaced. Even switching the adrenal glands back on.

Eye problems resolved that are caused by oxidative damage done by free radicals to the eye structures like the retina, lenses or circulatory system that feeds the eye. These problems being cured by nutritional support (the food God has given us) and giving the body lots of anti-oxidants. We don't need to do thousands of dollars of radiologic imaging and testing. We need to eliminate foods that cause oxidative damage to the tissues. Most times our bodies are just responding to inflammatory processes due to bad foods.

I sat in a doctor's office where people where not going through chemotherapy but nutritional support for cancer treatment.

I was reading about a Pastor that is well known whose daughter was dying of asthma in the hospital, a problem my grandson had trouble with also. They turned to naturopathic doctors who he had persuaded his doctors to let them try to treat her since she couldn't leave the hospital. They started treatment while she was there and these doctors gave her nutritional supplements. She walked out of the hospital shortly after.

I've heard that fasting, which most people just can't do or won't do and is suggested by God himself can heal our bodies. I think it's incredible after seeing what it did for my granddaughter. But I read that a prolonged fast, like what Jesus did can cause the body to detoxify itself to the point of turning on tumors and eating them. Now, that's incredible chemotherapy I think! Most impressive is the spiritual power and healing it produces as exemplified by Jesus and the great power he had after his fast. The holistic approach to healing is unspeakable.

So I want to encourage my readers to give God a chance as I did. Let him guide this, of course. What's important is that you don't miss this opportunity to see what God can do. "Oh taste and see that the LORD is good." Psalms 34:8

I just want to tell you what you can look forward to when

you enter the health care system of God. It is an exciting journey and its end is true wealth through health and prosperity. I had to step out on faith to experience it.

If you enjoyed reading this book, here's more books by the author:

1. Natural Cures for Perfect Health: Jesus Christ Will Cure You But the Doctor's Won't

http://amzn.to./2Dz23a0

2. Health Food Book, Detox Diet for Long Term Health

http://amzn.to/2pdf536

3. Aniya's Health and Food Book

http://amzn.to/2tnCi4b

4. Aaron's Preschool Book Fruits of the Spirit
http://amzn.to/2p4n5Hn

5. Aaron's Preschool Book For 3 Year Olds: A Little Boy's Adventures

http://amzn.to/2qzFgo5

6. Aaron and Aniya's Beginners Bible, A Children's First bible Book

http://amzn.to/2t5vCau

7. God's Health Care System, Receiving Healing Health Stories From The Holy Bible

http://amzn.to/2CYociL

About the Author:

Shelly Jenkins is a native of Chicago, Illinois and has been a believer in Christ since young adulthood. An avid bible scholar and bachelors prepared registered nurse for more than 32 years, she has worked in a variety of nursing areas including Maternal Child Health, Nursing Education, and Child Welfare Services. Currently a school nurse for over 10 years and legal nurse consultant, she has a passion for health, healing and wellness through a biblical perspective. An artist in her spare time, she is a mother of two and a grandmother of four and is currently living in Columbus, Ohio.

Shelly Jenkins

Email: shellyjenkins13@gmail.com

www.godshealthcaresystem.com